Renee Sommer
Simplicity & Meaning Coaching
Eau Claire WI 54703
www.reneesommer.com

Printed in the United States of America

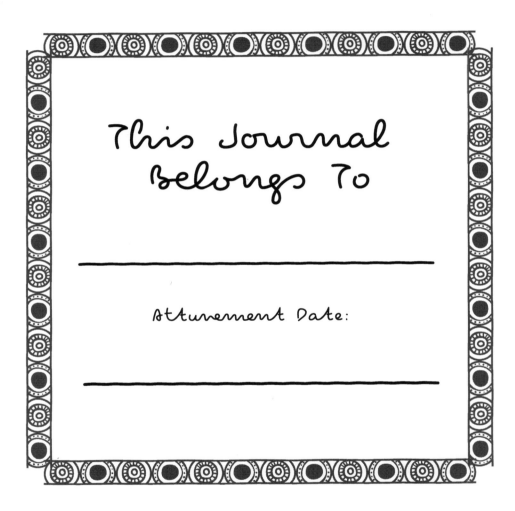

This Journal
Belongs To

_____

Attunement Date:

_____

Welcome!

This journal is meant to help you process the 21 days post Reiki attunement but can also be a great resource whenever you need to reconnect with your Reiki practice as well.

I'm very honored you chose to take your Reiki journey with me whether I'm your Reiki master or simply the creator of this journal for you.

Love & Light,
Renee Sommer

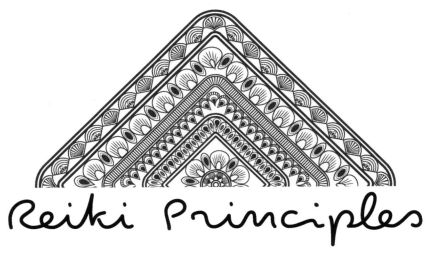

Reiki Principles

Just for today I will not worry.
Just for today I will not be angry.
Just for today I will do my work honestly.
Just for today I will give thanks for my many
blessings.
Just for today I will be kind to my neighbor and
every living thing.

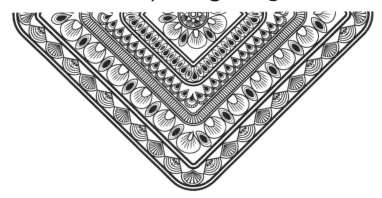

Habit Tracker

Track your daily treatments so you don't miss a single day (especially during your first 21 days!). You can use the rest to track additional months or other habits you'd like to incorporate for self-care such as a spiritual practice, pampering, water intake, etc.

Day	Self Treatments													
1														
2														
3														
4														
5														
6														
7														
8														
9														
10														
11														
12														
13														
14														
15														
16														
17														
18														
19														
20														
21														
22														
23														
24														
25														
26														
27														
28														
29														
30														
31														

Day 1: Describe your attunement experience and how you feel about your journey thus far.

_____

_____

_____

_____

_____

_____

_____

_____

_____

_____

_____

_____

_____

_____

_____

_____

_____

_____

_____

_____

Day 2: What doubts have you had about this experience so far?

Day 3: Think about your Reiki principles. What one feels like the biggest challenge?

Day 4: Have you felt any sort of shifts in your life recently?
Describe them below.

Day 5: What do you need to start saying YES to in your life?

Day 6: What do you need to start saying NO to in your life?

_____

_____

_____

_____

_____

_____

_____

_____

_____

_____

_____

_____

_____

_____

_____

_____

_____

_____

_____

_____

Day 7: What inspired you to begin this journey? How will it continue to guide you?

_____

_____

_____

_____

_____

_____

_____

_____

_____

_____

_____

_____

_____

_____

_____

_____

_____

_____

Day 8: One challenging area in my life is _____ and I hope
Reiki can help _____.

Day 9: How does Reiki tie into your sense of spirituality or your belief system?

_____

_____

_____

_____

_____

_____

_____

_____

_____

_____

_____

_____

_____

_____

_____

_____

_____

_____

_____

Day 10: Are you experiencing any energetic detox symptoms? Describe them or ponder why not below.

Day 11: Why was now the right time in your life for this journey?

_____

_____

_____

_____

_____

_____

_____

_____

_____

_____

_____

_____

_____

_____

_____

_____

_____

_____

_____

_____

Day 12: Describe your self-treatments so far. What have you experienced?

Day 13: Who inspires you most to show up more lovingly in the world?

Day 14: Just for today, I will not worry. What does this mean for you?

Day 15: Just for today, I will not be angry. How can you live this principle better in your life?

Day 16: Just for today, I will do my work honestly. What do you believe you were put here to accomplish?

Day 17: Just for today, I will give thanks for my many blessings. Make a list of 21 things you are thankful for.

Day 18: Just for today, I will be kind to every living thing. How could you apply this in your life more often?

_____

_____

_____

_____

_____

_____

_____

_____

_____

_____

_____

_____

_____

_____

_____

_____

_____

_____

_____

Day 19: Have you treated a friend or family member at this point? Why or why not? And if so, what did you experience?

Day 20: How has Reiki surprised you in the last 20 days?

Day 21: On this final day of transition, use the following pages to reflect on your journey, your doubts, your fears, and your hopes for the future.

Made in the USA
Coppell, TX
21 February 2025

46219729R00017